The Natural Diet

Simple Nutritional Advice For Optimal Health In The Modern World

Patrick Barrett

TABLE OF CONTENTS

"Tell me what you eat, and I will tell you who you are."

-Jean Anthelme Brillat-Savarin, 1755-1826
French lawyer, politician, epicure, gastronome

INTRODUCTION

Hello there!

First of all, I would like to thank you sincerely for purchasing this book. I know it means a lot to spend time and money on something, especially when you're hoping to learn something and improve yourself, and even more so when it comes to your health and well-being. Rest assured that I will do everything I can to make sure it's worth your while.

Now, allow me to introduce myself.

My name is Patrick Barrett. I am not a doctor or a dietitian. Although I have taken a few college courses on the subject, and I have read dozens (if not hundreds) of pertinent books, I am not certified in any way to teach people about nutrition. You should always talk to your doctor before taking advice on diet, nutrition, exercise, or your health in general, whether it comes from me or anybody else, and you should get his okay before making any health-related lifestyle changes.

Now that we've covered what I'm definitely not, here's what I am. I am a person who has been interested in health, exercise, and nutrition for as long as I can remember. I have studied (informally, on my own) the nutritional habits of elite athletes and ancient cultures. I have tried a variety of crazy dietary ideas out on myself, with a wide spectrum of results. I have looked into claims made by various nutritional 'authorities' (government agencies and big food companies, for example) and been shocked by what I found out.

In the beginning I would jump from one nutritional philosophy to another, but I always had a nagging feeling that what I was trying... just didn't make any sense. Have you ever had that feeling? Some magazine or book or guy on TV says "This list of foods is good for you, and this list is bad. Always do this, and never do that." Meanwhile, one person's list looks completely different from someone else's, and what 'everybody' is saying you should eat is the exact opposite of what 'everybody' said you should eat ten years ago, which is completely different from what was 'in' another ten years before that.

The other aspect is that, on an intuitive level, these diet fads just don't make sense.

Some people say milk and dairy are bad for us. How can milk be bad, if we're mammals, and milk is sufficiently nutritious to feed us through the period of our lives when good nutrition is most critical?

Other authorities will insist that the only way to be healthy is to eat a more or less flavorless diet. How can a 'healthy' diet be so unpleasant to the senses—in other words, why would our noses and tongues make 'unhealthy' food seem appealing, and 'healthy' bland and undesirable?

Still others will tell you that you must take some supplement or eat some invented superfood for optimal health. How can our bodies 'require' a certain food product that has only been created in recent history? Were human beings never healthy until its invention, and did the human body somehow evolve to require a product that didn't even exist yet? So many of the most common ideas in nutrition just don't hold up if you spend a few minutes thinking about them.

Couple this with the fact that there are cultures all around the world who spend no time thinking about being fat or thin and enjoy longer lives and better health than most in the developed West do, and it becomes clear that we're missing something important on an intuitive level.

I don't claim to have all the answers to every question, but I can say that after years of trial and error with one approach after another, I have had the best personal results by ignoring, or just breaking, most of the mainstream rules that we've all heard about when it comes to personal health and nutrition—and I've come up with some guidelines of my own that make sense and get results.

In this book, I have sought to summarize all the most important parts of more than a decade of my nutritional pursuits, and to condense all the most important recommendations and warnings I can offer into a resource that the average person can read through and absorb without years of wasting time or studying terminology. My goal is to clear up some of the misconceptions out there which, I believe, are the cause of a lot of physical and emotional pain and discomfort for a lot of people.

I hope you find it to be valuable.

Books by Patrick Barrett:

Natural Exercise: Basic Bodyweight Training and Calisthenics for Strength and Weight-Loss

The Natural Diet: Simple Nutritional Advice For Optimal Health In The Modern World

BEFORE WE GET STARTED

By the time you reach the end of this book, you'll be able to form an opinion on the things I've told you. Between now and then, though, it would be best if you tried to approach everything I'm going to say with a clean slate. Some ideas will go completely against major tenets of mainstream nutrition. Some are just ways of looking at food that you've probably never heard of or seen before. In either case, it's best if, at least for the duration of the book, you forget what you've heard before and just worry about whether or not what I'm saying makes any sense to you.

Also, please (not just in this book, but in general) don't decide whether or not something is true based on how many other people think it's true. History is full of examples of brilliant people who developed new (and correct) ideas that were rejected by everybody. Galileo wasn't less right about the planets because everybody was against him. I'm not saying this book is an event of that magnitude, of course, but the fact remains that there is plenty of evidence that large groups of people can be very wrong about very important things for a very long time.

Let's consider a few strange circumstances to be observed in the modern world, and particularly the United States, when it comes to nutrition.

* We spend a huge amount of time, money, and energy on diet books, DVDs, foods, trends, magazines, etc., yet we seem to have worsening rates of obesity, cancer, and heart disease each year.
* Many European and Asian countries spend much less time worrying about nutrition, but still tend to be much leaner and healthier.
* We all seem to know people who 'break all the rules' when it comes to food, yet they don't gain weight or suffer from ill health.
* Conversely, we all know people who 'do everything right' but can't seem to lose any weight at all, and often gain weight despite their efforts.

Doesn't it seem a little unreasonable that people who 'follow all the rules' can't seem to get anywhere? Doesn't that indicate that those rules probably aren't right?

For now, let's just agree that there does appear to be evidence that, as a group, we are on the wrong track when it comes to understanding what type of food is best for our bodies, and what needs to be avoided.

To resolve this situation, we'll need to do two things: first, we need to correct what we've heard so far, and sort out the good from the bad. Next, we need to learn to critically evaluate the information we receive in the future so that we know what we can trust—after all, much of the information that we learn about the 'benefits' of different foods comes from the people who sell us those foods. Remember that studies cost money, and companies won't spend that money unless they can use it to sell their products—not all such studies are privately funded, but many are, one way or another.

So if you're ready for it, let's get started right off the bat with the first section, which covers the pitfalls of 'nutrition facts.'

NUTRITION FACTS—WHAT AN ODD NAME

I know that we're going to talk about a lot of different topics which will go against what you're used to hearing. To get the ball rolling, we're going to start out by talking about one of the most basic and fundamental concepts of mainstream nutrition that everyone just takes for granted: namely, nutrition facts.

In this chapter, we're going to find out:

1. Why it is impossible to count calories, grams of anything, etc.,
2. Why there's no reason to count them in the first place.

The first thing we should talk about is the fact that, contrary to their portrayal, Nutrition Facts are not handed down by God. They are based on rules set forth by the United States Government. In other words, they are the work of a group of people who hired some other people to figure out some numbers for them a few decades ago. For most of human history there were no Nutrition Facts stamped on the side of food, and so far there's no real reason to believe that we're better off now that we have them.

These numbers are regulated by the FDA. Let's get into how that works, and you'll see how loose a term 'regulated' is in this context.

First and foremost, all numbers on the Nutrition Facts label are allowed to be off by 20 percent. That means that your 2,000 calories a day could really be 2,400 calories a day, and that's fine with the FDA. Twenty percent is a lot. What if you were suddenly 20 percent fatter? Or 20 percent leaner? What if you lost or gained twenty percent of your wealth? It makes a difference.

In case you don't believe me, here's the URL to the page on the FDA website that lays out these guidelines:

http://www.fda.gov/Food/GuidanceComplianceRegulatory Information/GuidanceDocuments/FoodLabelingNutrition/ ucm063113.htm

(You can also search the page title, "Nutrition Labeling Manual - A Guide for Developing and Using Data Bases" on Google. It should be the first result.)

Now if you know any of those people who live and die by the numbers of calories or grams of whatever they eat each day, or if you are one yourself, then this might be a pretty big shock to you. Well, then you need to get ready, because the next thing I say will be even more of a shock:

No one double-checks those numbers. the FDA does not analyze any food to find out how many calories or how many grams of fat, carbs, protein, or anything else it contains. The cost to analyze one food product can run well into six figures, so there's no way the FDA could reasonably check everything. So what do they do? Well, instead of checking everything themselves, the FDA simply trusts the company that produces the food to use whatever method they want to determine the nutrient values for the nutrition facts label.

Here's the quote from the page mentioned above:

"Although FDA encourages industry to submit nutrition labeling data bases to the agency for review, submission of a data base to FDA for the purpose of nutrition labeling is voluntary. The agency has not and does not intend to prescribe how an individual company is to determine nutrient content for labeling purposes."

Once those values are determined, however they are determined, the company can just send the report to the FDA, who files it away somewhere without verifying anything (again, they really can't verify all of that information). Then the company just produces that product with the information they say their scientists found. The only way the FDA will get involved or verify anything is if a lot of people complain, and there's some significant reason to believe the information is bad—and it takes a LOT of complaints to get the FDA to do anything it doesn't want to.

Take a second to think about all the low-calorie, low-carb, diet, lite, reduced fat, reduced sugar, etc., etc., products on the market today. In many cases people only buy those foods because of the nutritional claims.

Now think about the fact that companies have a huge monetary incentive to create delicious 'diet' snack food, and nobody really checks to see if what they claim, as far as nutritional content, is true.

What this all boils down to is that it isn't possible to know how many calories you eat, how many grams of protein you consume, how many carbs you have in a day, or anything else like that. I'll repeat that—it is not possible (okay, maybe it's almost possible with an unlimited budget, but it's not remotely practical). So where does that leave us?

Don't worry. The fact is that 'calories' and 'grams' are not a useful way to measure food. The standard line is that the average person should eat 2,000 calories a day (you can get a slightly more specific official number according to your demographics, but we'll say 2,000 for the sake of argument). That kind of value is absurd in the first place, but we'll ignore that for now.

Well, 2,000 calories could mean a gigantic bowl of fruit, or a few pounds of bacon, or more than a half gallon of ketchup. Or, it could mean any of an infinite number of combinations of other things. Eating these different daily intakes could produce any range of results, from an Olympic level physique to probable death within a few weeks. The fact that they all add up to the same number of calories is totally irrelevant.

Imagine that you need some parts to fix your car. Do you just order 30 pounds of car parts? Of course not. You need specific parts for specific purposes, and measuring those parts by weight isn't helpful. Similarly, your body craves certain nutrients, minerals, etc., and discussing them in terms of their caloric value is pointless.

This doesn't mean that you can eat an unlimited number of calories without concern—it is, of course, quite possible to overeat, and there's never a reason to stuff yourself intentionally—but in general it is much more important to focus on the quality of your food over the quantity. You should never feel bad about eating any reasonable amount of wholesome, fresh foods, but if you regularly eat so much that you feel stuffed, you can expect to have trouble losing weight and staying healthy.

The same principle about tracking calories goes for tracking grams of carbohydrates, fats, or proteins. 50g of sugar from strawberries has a completely different effect compared to 50g of sugar from a soda. Similarly, 15g of soy protein compared to 15g of beef protein is not at all the same. The same goes for 15g of margarine compared to 15g of coconut oil, and so on. In all of these cases, what is crucial is an understanding of what each of these foods does for your body, not what their masses are. Of course, we will discuss all of these things in the coming chapters.

While we're on the subject, I might as well point out that the measures of vitamins and minerals on Nutrition Facts are also not nearly as helpful as you might think. The usability of a vitamin or mineral varies extremely depending on where it comes from. Calcium that is found naturally in a food is infinitely more useful than another type of calcium which is isolated and then artificially added to a food. For that reason, two different foods that both claim to contain 25% of your daily recommended calcium intake will have two totally different results as far as calcium that your body can actually absorb and use. Also, calcium citrate and calcium carbonate, for example, can both be called 'calcium,' but your body handles them in two different ways. Similar statements can be made about other vitamins and minerals.

So what does it all mean? Is it impossible to know how much of which foods you should eat? Do you need to learn about every single incarnation of every single vitamin and mineral so that you can spend hours researching everything that goes into your mouth? No, and no. The resolution of these problems is actually very simple and intuitive, and we will discuss it all in the coming chapters.

FATS

If there is one misunderstood nutrient, it is fat.

We just talked about how Nutrition "Facts" are not facts at all. That's pretty big news to a lot of people, because it means that lots of big companies, our government, and dieters everywhere are spending a ton of time and money on something that is ultimately, well, not helpful. If that comes as a surprise, you'd better get used to it, because there's more coming.

In this chapter we'll be discussing the role of fat in your diet, and what you hear may surprise you. Fat is incredibly important in your body. It is absolutely vital for good health, particularly for athletes. Vitamins A, E, D, and K are fat-soluble, which means you can only consume them in fat. Bottom line—you need fat.

This is the part where you expect me to say "It is important to eat healthy fats, but only in moderation." I'm not going to. You might also expect me to say "Be sure to consume heart-healthy vegetable oils and stay away from saturated fats." Wrong again.

Remember how we talked about Nutrition Facts? Well, one of my college professors was one of the nutritionists who helped determine which information should be listed among those facts, as well as which magic numbers people should aim for. He informed us that the recommended daily intake was already based on a low-fat diet. Now, remember, fat is very important to your body, and these nutritionists built a diet which is already low in fat to begin with, and many people take that diet and eliminate even more fat from it (and then are mystified when their bodies don't seem to respond well).

So I raised my hand and asked "If that diet is already low-fat, what would be a normal level of fat intake?" Get ready for this.

He said that the ideal normal level of fat intake was "maybe fifty, fifty-five percent of calories from fat." That's compared to the 30% they recommend.

I'm not saying I necessarily agree with those numbers exactly—in fact, I don't even really think about it in those terms. But here's a nutritionist who helped determine how much fat the government recommends you eat, and he freely admits that the ideal amount is nearly twice as much.

The key to proper fat consumption is eating only natural fats. We'll talk more later about what 'natural' really means in general, but in order to talk about what natural fats are, we'll talk about how the bad seed oils are produced.

When I say bad seed oils, I am primarily talking about soybean oil (sold as "vegetable oil") and rape oil (sold as "canola oil"), and just about anything else from a seed (there are some exceptions, we'll get into that).

First, the seeds are ground up into a kind of pulp. The first problem is separating the oil from the shell. That is done by mixing in hexane, a mild anesthetic found in gasoline and heavy-duty glues. The hexane separates the oils from the shells, but then you're left with a mixture of seed oil and hexane. A centrifuge is used to remove most—but not all—of the hexane. What you are left with is seed oil with a small percentage of hexane—that soon smells horrible, because it is decomposing (that's not a typo).

You know how people are always talking about how great unsaturated fat is? Well, polyunsaturated fat—like what you find in seeds—is incredibly unstable, and once it's out of that seed and exposed to heat, light, and air, it starts to decompose. You know, rot.

So those oils smell pretty awful. They're not going to sell too well like that. In order to take care of that, the oils are then sprayed with super-heated steam for a long time until everything that smells is burnt away. Then there is no smell, or flavor, at all. That's why those vegetable oils don't smell or taste like anything (doesn't 'not smelling or tasting like anything' sound like it should be a warning sign anyway?).

That's how vegetable oils are produced. In case it hasn't struck you yet, this does not fall into the category of a natural fat. As a general rule, if you need a whole factory to make something, it isn't natural.

Want to know how olive oil, peanut oil, and coconut oil are made? Crush olives, peanuts, or coconut meat, and collect the oil that comes out. That's it. Obviously today these are also produced in factories, but that's just for greater efficiency. If you wanted to you could still get the oil out using two big, flat rocks and nothing else.

That's an example of natural fat. These fats are stable enough not to decompose (although ideally they should still be kept away from light and heat), so they don't have to be sprayed and deodorized, which is why olive oil smells like olives, peanut oil smells like peanuts, and coconut oil smells like coconuts. A good rule of thumb is that any fat or oil you consume should smell like what it is —no odor or flavor is a bad, bad sign.

Other natural fats include butter, duck fat, and other animal fats. They are all highly stable, all largely saturated, and all natural.

I know, I just said butter and animal fats were good for you, which instantly puts me on some kind of dietary blacklist for some people. But consider the fact that Americans have eaten steadily less butter and more bad seed oils in the past hundred years, and heart disease and obesity rates have all gotten worse. Just a thought.

I know a lot of people are going to feel uncomfortable with animal fats, and if you do, there's always olive, peanut, coconut, or any other oil that actually tastes like something. Personally I always default to butter, but I use olive, peanut, and coconut oils as well.

The key to eating healthy fat is eliminating the unnatural, unstable, damaged fats, and sticking to the whole, healthy, intact ones. At this point it should go without saying, but stay far away from margarines or 'spreads' made from unnatural vegetable oils. These are extremely processed, extremely damaged, and extremely unhealthy.

Don't fear fat. You need it. Stop buying skim milk, reduced fat cheese, and fat-free yogurt. Get your dairy as close to natural as possible, which means full fat and no additives (get plain whole-fat yogurt and add flavor with raw honey and/or chopped fruit, if you like—it's healthier and tastes better anyway).

Since we've been talking about fats, this is probably a good time to discuss cholesterol.

We think of cholesterol as very unhealthy, but if you had no cholesterol in your body, you would die very quickly.

Cholesterol is a sterol produced by your body that is vital to the proper functioning of cell membranes. Most of the cholesterol in your body is there not because you ate it, but because your body went out of its way to make it—because it's important.

People are very scared of cholesterol, but the aura of danger surrounding it is very poorly founded. For example, many cultures eat tons of cholesterol and have healthy hearts, such as the French, the Germans, and the Masai. In fact, studies that show ill effects because of cholesterol are hard to replicate outside of the United States.

If someone has a high level of blood cholesterol, eating less cholesterol probably won't help because your body fights hard to maintain its cholesterol levels, and in fact recent studies have shown that an increased cholesterol intake will lead to decreased cholesterol production in your body, while decreasing cholesterol intake causes your body to increase production.

Some researches have theorized that cholesterol in your blood is not actually unhealthy, but can be an indicator of other health problems, and decreasing the cholesterol level in your blood does not impact the root cause of the problem in any way.

Cholesterol is a substance that your body goes out of its way to produce that is vital to cell membranes, acts as an antioxidant, and is associated with proper uptake of serotonin (which affects mood and digestion). Many cultures including the Masai warriors, the Samburu, the French, and others consume and have long consumed relatively large quantities without any ill effects to heart health or other health (and in at least the case of the Masai, there is evidence of incredible physical health). I eat a lot of cholesterol and don't give it a thought. While there is a lot of evidence to support the idea that cholesterol is not bad for you and is even an important part of a healthy diet, there is a multi-billion dollar drug industry which says it is a big problem, and people need expensive daily medication to fight it.

I'm not a doctor, and you should never stop taking any medication without talking to one, but I do think there is more than one side to the cholesterol story, and I encourage you to look into and discuss it with your doctor if you feel the need.

Resources:

The Coconut Oil Miracle
By Bruce Fife and Jon J. Kabara

This book focuses on coconut oil—which is pretty amazing stuff—but also provides a good primer on fats in general. You'll find out a lot you never knew about what's really good about the good fats, and what's really bad about the bad ones.

Ignore the Awkward: How the Cholesterol Myths Are Kept Alive
By Dr. Uffe Ravnskov

Dr. Ravnskov is a longtime skeptic of the mainstream cholesterol hypothesis, and this book gives a good explanation as to why.

INTACT NUTRIENTS

The biggest health consequence of the modern lifestyle, and one of the least understood problems facing people in developed, industrial countries, is the scarcity of intact nutrients. Let's talk about what that means.

Imagine that you order a beautiful crystal vase on eBay. You live in New York and it's shipping from California. Imagine that the shipper just throws it in the box without wrapping it in newspaper, or packing it in anything. By the time it makes the cross country trip, what you receive instead of a crystal vase is a box full of crystal shards. It doesn't matter how beautiful it was when it was put in there if it's shattered by the time it gets to you.

This situation illustrates the problem with processed foods. Many of the vitamins, enzymes (we'll talk about them in a minute), proteins, etc., that your body needs are pretty fragile. In order to get the maximum benefit of, for example, vitamin C, you need to get it, more or less, straight out of the orange (or wherever else it came from).

If you drink pasteurized orange juice (which almost all commercially available orange juice is), the vitamin C is severely damaged if not completely useless. It doesn't matter that when the orange was juiced at the factory it was full of vitamin C, because by the time it gets cooked (pasteurized) and exposed to heat, light, and air in the processing and shipping process, it's useless to your body. That's why fresh orange juice will actually fight a cold, and 'normal' orange juice actually makes it worse.

I used vitamin C as an example, but the same is true of an untold number of other nutrients. The more cooking and processing food goes through, the more the nutrients it contains become denatured, damaged, and useless.

Let's talk briefly about antioxidants. Antioxidants neutralize free radicals. Free radicals cause damaging chain reactions by oxidizing one molecule, which in turn becomes a free radical and oxidizes its neighbor, and so on and so on. That chain reaction stops once it hits an antioxidant, which is able to get oxidized and then stop the process. Any specific antioxidant molecule can only do this one time. When antioxidants are exposed to air, they get oxidized and become useless. This is what you see when you cut an apple in half and leave it on the counter and it turns brown. It also happens to orange juice once it gets squeezed out of an orange, and to almost any other fresh food when its insides are exposed to air.

In general, when you take an antioxidant away from its natural context, it gets oxidized and becomes useless. That's why you shouldn't count on antioxidants in pasteurized foods, and you shouldn't believe it when a food product has added antioxidants, because isolating antioxidants from one source so they can be added to something else is going to expose them to a lot of light, heat, and air, and almost certainly ruin them.

Some of you might be saying to yourselves, "well how can they say that there are added antioxidants in a food if the antioxidants are useless?" If you are one of those people, I think you might have slept through the chapter on Nutrition Facts, but the bottom line is that the people who regulate such things are either not knowledgeable enough, or just don't care enough to make such distinctions. A big part of what the FDA does is to help make it possible for big food companies to sell food and make money, and making positive claims about added antioxidants is just one of those nonsensical things the FDA is okay with.

Anyway, let's get back on track. The good news here is that you don't need to learn about every single class of nutrient and every single specific example of each class, and exactly how and when they break down. All you really need to know is that the more processed and cooked something is, the more damaged it is, and when someone artificially adds a vitamin or antioxidant or other nutrient to a product in order to make it seem more healthy, it doesn't mean much because it's probably pretty useless by the time it gets into your body. Still, it's useful to talk in general about some of the amazing things in uncooked, unprocessed foods that are lost in the cooking and processing, so let's do that.

Enzymes

Enzymes are amazing little delicate proteins found in all raw, natural foods that help your body to digest those foods. For example, unpasteurized milk has the enzyme lactase, which works specifically on the sugar that is found in milk (lactose).

Enzymes are so amazing because they're like little helpers built right into food so that when you start to digest it, it helps your body out and pretty much does the digestion for you. If not for the enzymes already found in food, digestion would be an incredibly tiring and difficult process for your body to go through, and every time you ate a big meal you would get really really tired from the effort of digestion. Hold on a second—people do get really tired after big meals! What's up with that?

Well, the thing about enzymes is they break down somewhere between 118 and 140 degrees Fahrenheit. That means anything you eat that has been pasteurized or cooked contains basically no functional enzymes—which is why Thanksgiving dinner leaves everyone exhausted, and why most people have trouble staying awake for a little while after lunch. That tired feeling you get after eating a lot isn't supposed to be a part of the digestive process—but it is, largely because the foods people eat contain few or no working enzymes.

An example I always like to use for this is eggs. With some frequency I'll blend up six eggs with some unpasteurized milk and raw honey in my blender. Afterward I feel very energized—not tired at all. If I were to take just those six eggs and cook them into an omelet, and eat that instead—I'd want to head right back to bed. It's so much more difficult for your body to digest something when you've destroyed it with heat or processing.

Uncooked and unprocessed foods are incredibly energizing and nourishing for your body. That doesn't mean everything you eat has to be raw, or that you have to consume any raw meat, eggs, or dairy at all if you aren't comfortable with that. However, for optimal health you must consume fresh fruit—whatever kind you like, however much you like, as long as it's fresh (apples, not applesauce; an orange, not a container of mandarin orange slices in syrup, and so on).

We'll discuss the benefits of fruit in greater detail later, but I wanted to clarify the 'raw' thing. Raw fruit is an ideal fuel for your body, and if you don't make it a major component of your diet, you'll never be optimally healthy.

Raw food is whole, natural, undamaged, and useful nutrient-rich. It is exactly what your body is made to digest and handle. Cooked food is denatured, damaged, and useful nutrient-poor. It forces your body to waste a lot of unnecessary time and energy on more difficult digestion. I'm not saying you can't eat cooked food and be healthy, but an understanding of the differences between cooked food and uncooked food is vital to good health.

P.S.

I just wanted to add something at the end here so we can talk about pasteurization and what it means to you. You probably know that pasteurization is a process by which foods are exposed to a certain degree of heat for a certain amount of time in order to kill bacteria and theoretically make the food safer to consume. Many foods are pasteurized, most notably dairy products, but also fruit juices, products containing eggs, and other foods.

Pasteurization does generally kill bacteria, but the heat also destroys enzymes and damages untold other nutrients. This has the overall effect of making the food 'safer' in terms of bacteria but less healthy in terms of nutrients.

Pasteurization was developed at a time when options for shipping and storage of food were not nearly as advanced as they are now. It afforded a lot of products which would otherwise have gone bad, and been unsellable, a longer shelf life, which increased profits for food producers.

Today, pasteurization is basically a cheaper alternative to fresh food. It is entirely possible to deliver raw milk fresh to any grocery store, but it is more expensive and most people don't know the difference (and in many states it is illegal, which is another story). It is entirely possible to juice oranges and other fruits in the store and sell them immediately, and some stores do this, but in general it is more expensive and not enough people know the difference to increase the demand and lower the price.

So, whereas most people think of pasteurization as a good thing, I think of it as a bad thing, and when I mention pasteurized food, I mean it's something you should avoid if fresher options are available.

For example, fresh fruit juice (like juice that you make in your home or that someone makes with a juicer right in front of you) is healthy and should be consumed as often as you like, but store-bought pasteurized fruit juice is not much better than sugar water, and should for the most part be treated the same as soda or any other artificial, processed sugar-laden drink. More on fruit in the next chapter.

FRUIT

Let's talk for a little bit about fruit. In the last chapter I told you about the importance of consuming nutrients in their natural state, because when they are processed or isolated they are damaged. Well, the all-time greatest source of vitamins, enzymes, raw carbohydrates, and tons of other good stuff is fresh fruit.

Basically, fruit is exactly what your body is made to eat. Carnivores, like lions, have relatively short digestive tracts for digesting raw meat. It's not so hard to digest raw meat because it is nutrient-dense and easily assimilated. Herbivores, like cows, have very long digestive tracts, because it takes a lot of digesting to get much nutrition out of grass and similar plants. Omnivores, like people, have a medium-length digestive tract which is pretty good at digesting meat and pretty good at digesting vegetation—but best at digesting fruit.

Chimpanzees, whose digestive tracts are a lot like ours, eat the majority of their diet as fruit. You don't have to eat the majority of your diet as fruit (although it's probably not a bad idea), but aiming for at least a third to a half of your diet as fresh fruit is a good goal.

You are made to eat fruit. This is where the constant cravings for sweets comes from—your body is craving the natural sugars found in fresh ripe fruit! However, since most people are used to satisfying that sweet craving with candy, or pastries, or who knows what else, they never make this connection. Also, since your body never gets what it craves, the craving never goes away.

I'm not saying that this knowledge alone will eradicate any craving you have for unnatural and unhealthy foods, but it can help you to reduce them significantly in less time than you think, which is something we'll cover more in the chapter on cravings.

The amount of disease people deal with in the industrialized world is not at all surprising when you consider that many people consume no fresh fruit on a regular basis. If you want to be healthy, you need to make fresh fruit a large and regular part of your diet. A variety is good, but if your favorite fruit is apples and you mainly eat those, that's totally fine. Get used to going to the store at least a couple of times a week and keeping fresh fruit on hand—again, whichever fruit you like the most, just eat it regularly.

I'll just take this opportunity to remind you that I'm only talking about fresh fruit. Something that says "made with 100% fruit" or "contains real fruit!" does not count. Something can be made out of only strawberries, but if they are mashed up and cooked down and filtered and oxidized and who knows what else, they are still 100% fruit, but they are definitely not fresh. If something is really fresh fruit, you can tell, because it will just be a piece of fruit and not require any further claims or explanation. Other than that, don't fall for it.

P.S.

Frozen fruit is okay. Nothing is better than fresh, but if you are (for example) going to make a smoothie, and you have frozen berries (I mean berries that were picked and frozen without any further additives or processing), then that is pretty close to fresh, and you shouldn't worry so much about it—freezing is a much less destructive process than cooking is in this situation, although as always, fresh is best.

ANIMAL PRODUCTS

There are many people who hear about a 'raw food diet' and think that means a vegetarian or vegan diet. Since the diet I recommend is partially raw, I want to make sure that you understand that I absolutely recommend consuming animal products as well.

Meat

People have eaten meat for quite a long time, and anthropologists connect the beginning of higher brain function with the start of people consuming meat (in large part due to fats and cholesterol). Anthropologists also find that tribes that make animal products an important part of their diets are healthier, stronger, and more dominant than neighboring tribes who subsist on vegetation and roots (the Masai are a great example of this).

There have been studies that connect meat with a variety of diseases and death, but those studies often suffer from some major flaws, the greatest of which is they make no distinction between thoroughly processed and additive-laden meats (like most commercially available bacon, sausage, salami, cold cuts, and meats found in frozen foods) and fresh, unprocessed, lightly cooked meats, which is kind of like saying there's no difference between drinking spring water and drinking chlorinated pool water, since they're both water.

Many studies that proclaim that meat causes cancer and other problems are funded by groups backed by animal rights activists or similar organizations—just as there are a lot of studies with marketing motivation behind them, there are also politically-motivated studies. I'm not saying any study you find is worthless, but I am saying that before you accept any findings, find out which group did the study and where that group got its money. That way, you'll have a better idea whether the primary motivation of the researcher was to answer a question accurately, or to provide ammo for a political agenda. That's a good policy to follow whether you're finding out about a study related to nutrition, or to anything else.

Also, it is generally very difficult to prove a negative relationship between meat consumption and health in studies outside of the United States and the developed West, probably because food consumed in the U.S. is generally much more processed and denatured than food found in many other parts of the world.

This is actually the tip of a very interesting iceberg—very often similar nutritional studies, meat-related or otherwise, done in different countries will report very different findings, which suggests that a combination of bias among researchers and a poor understanding of what really matters in nutrition is leading to bad research. Along the same lines, many different cultures have completely different commonly accepted ideas of what constitutes healthy and unhealthy eating.

Fish

My advice on fish is similar to my advice on meat—eat it. Wild-caught is much better than farmed (farmed fish contains lots of added hormones and other bad stuff), and the more lightly cooked, the better.

Dairy

Dairy has also been a major part of the human diet for a long time, and I would definitely recommend that you make it a part of your diet (although it's not absolutely required, if you don't like it). I would make a couple of recommendations, though.

1. Eat full fat. Don't get reduced fat cheese or fat-free yogurt. The fat is an important part of the food, and it's not good to avoid it.
2. Pick additive-free dairy. If it contains more than some combination of milk, cream, salt, rennet, and some kind of starter culture, I wouldn't buy it.
3. Choose dairy that's either raw (unpasteurized) or cultured (like yogurt, some butter, and sour cream).

The vast majority of lactose-intolerant people have no trouble with raw dairy. All milk and cheeses which have been pasteurized will say so on the package somewhere. Some cheese will state in its ingredients it is made with either "raw," "unpasteurized," or "fresh" milk, but even if it just says "milk" and doesn't say anywhere that it's been pasteurized, then it's raw.

There is lactose in raw milk, just as in pasteurized milk, but there is also lactase, the enzyme that breaks down lactose. All the lactase in pasteurized milk is destroyed in the pasteurization process, which can make it difficult to digest for some people. If you have trouble with dairy, you may want to experiment (with small amounts at first, of course) with raw milk and see if it gives you any trouble.

As a side note, I have noticed that organic pasteurized milk seems to be significantly easier to digest than conventional pasteurized milk. To be honest, I don't really know why that would be, but I can say from personal experience that there is a difference, and although organic pasteurized is not as good as raw milk, it's a passable alternative that is worth your consideration.

Personally, I eat a lot of whole-fat plain yogurt (I either use it to make a smoothie, or mix in honey and fruit and have a bowl of it) and a lot of raw cheese. I drink milk if it's raw (and sometimes pasteurized organic), and generally when I cook something, I use butter. Also I make my own whole-fat sour cream-based dressings.

Having said all of that, I'll repeat again that I don't feel that dairy is an absolute necessity to a healthy diet per se, but it can be an important part of one.

Eggs

Eggs are a fantastic food. Contrary to popular belief, it is the yolk, and not the white, which contains all of the nutrients, and the runnier you can stand to eat it, the better. Often, I just put raw egg yolks into smoothies and throw the rest of the egg away.

Look at it this way. That little white piece attached to the yolk is the embryonic chicken. The yolk is what it feeds off to get its nutrients and grow—in other words, the yolk contains everything necessary to build a whole chicken. The white is just the clear stuff that the chicken and the yolk float in—there's some protein in there, but otherwise there's not much to it.

If you're going to eat an egg raw, only eat the yolk—the white contains some nutrients which should only be eaten cooked, so eat the white cooked or not at all.

Soy

Most people who avoid animal products turn to soy. I would strongly discourage this. Soy-based foods, especially those that are commonly commercially available outside of Asia, are some of the most processed and damaged foods available. Just look at how long the list of ingredients is on a soy-protein bar or soy-based meat substitute. You don't want any part of that. You could write a whole book on what's wrong with soy (people have), but suffice it to say that whatever good you've heard about it isn't true, or is at least very misleading.

Soybeans contain anti-nutrients and enzyme inhibitors, so they must be fermented even to be consumable. American soy products are not fermented because it is a time-consuming process, so all of those bad things are still intact.

Asians do not eat nearly as much soy as we imagine (although they are beginning to eat more now because marketers have told them that we in the West do). When they do eat soy, they generally eat traditional, fermented, painstakingly-created soy foods unlike anything we have in America.

Soy was popularized in America by 20th century industrialists like Henry Ford who were not healthy and who saw soy as a business opportunity (which has proven to be extremely lucrative). Ford tried to connect soy to the famous longevity enjoyed by Okinawans, who were actually shown in studies to consume more calories from pork than from any other food, and to only eat traditional Japanese soy foods that were vastly different from soy foods sold in America.

The soy craze of the past few years does seem to be cooling rapidly now that people have had more exposure to it, but soy and soy-based ingredients are everywhere, so check your labels and avoid it wherever possible. The only soy product I would recommend eating is fermented soy sauce.

Honorable Mention: Beans And Lentils

These aren't animal products of course, but as a good source of protein they deserve a mention. Beans and lentils have a lot of nutritional value, and the good news is that they are frequently available canned without any real additives to worry about. If you're not as into eating meat, or if you're just looking for variety, (non-soy) beans and lentils are definitely worth a look.

Animal products are an important part of the human diet. If you don't want to eat meat, I would absolutely recommend consuming unpasteurized and/or cultured dairy, and eggs as runny as you can stand them, as well as beans and lentils (beans and lentils must be fully cooked for your body to be able to use them). When you eat meat or fish you certainly don't have to eat it raw, but I would recommend cooking it as lightly as you're comfortable with and NOT avoiding the fat (you may be surprised by how much you like this if you aren't used to it).

Don't eat soy products disguised as meat. They are completely unnatural. Furthermore, avoid in general any kind of food that has been processed to taste and feel like another kind of food (turkey 'bacon' comes to mind). In order to accomplish this 'miracle of modern science,' the original food is usually heavily processed.

Resources:

The Whole Soy Story: The Dark Side of America's Favorite Health Food
By Kaayla T. Daniel

Understanding the media and marketing phenomenon of soy products is key to understanding the current state of health that America is in. You will be amazed when you find out the history of this food 'movement,' and you'll learn a lot along the way about a variety of associated nutritional concepts.

The Untold Story of Milk: The History, Politics and Science of Nature's Perfect Food
By Ron Schmid

This book will shed some light on dairy, another controversial part of the modern diet. Learn the compelling argument in favor of raw dairy, and the peculiar political history behind it.

GRAINS

One of the first things anybody remotely involved in the 'health food' scene for the past few decades will say to you is you have to eat fiber and whole grains to be healthy.

You don't, actually.

The fact is that grains are a completely unnecessary part of the human diet. Think about it. It's not possible for you to pick a grain and eat it. If you were a 'wild' human being, grains couldn't be a part of your diet, because grains can't be effectively digested by people without being processed and/or cooked in some way.

Who can eat grains? Cows, horses, sheep... what do we have in common with them from a digestive standpoint? Not much.

I know bread has been a huge and important part of the human diet for millenia. But why was bread always such a big deal? Because growing grains to make bread created a reliable source of food, not necessarily a highly nutritive one—and, of course, bread made hundreds of years ago was much more natural and less processed than the bread you get today.

Making bread is easier and more stable than hunting or raising animals, so bread has always been important. In the modern world that's not such a concern.

It is, of course, absolutely possible to eat grains and be healthy. There are plenty of healthy people who eat grain products every day, but your body doesn't require them in any amount. You can get plenty of carbohydrates (and all the fiber you need) from fruit, beans, and vegetables. If you're going to eat them, then of course the less processed they are the better, but I would keep them to a minimum, and you should definitely never feel compelled to add them to your diet.

WHAT DOES NATURAL MEAN?

I advocate not just 'a' natural diet, but 'the' natural human diet, or as close as you can come to it. I can't possibly claim that the way I eat or recommend that you eat is itself the one and only natural human diet, especially because diet varies for people all over the world, but it is certainly much closer than the vast majority of what people in the modern world eat, and I believe that eating 'the' natural diet should absolutely be your goal if you want to be as healthy as possible.

You've probably heard that before, though. "Eat natural." Why is this different?

Well, 'natural' has become something of a marketing buzzword in the food industry. Unlike terms such as 'low fat,' 'diet,' and 'organic,' 'natural' has no technical definition or qualifications, so really pretty much anybody can use it to describe anything. If anything, 'natural' has come to mean that a product's packaging uses earth tones, and you are expected to pay a little extra for it. That doesn't really help us.

The word 'natural' has become a distorted term for use in marketing. Don't accept anyone else's definition of natural, and don't believe any company that describes its own product as natural until you've had a look at the ingredients.

The ingredients in truly natural food come directly, physically (not chemically) out of the ground or an animal. Generally speaking, natural ingredients are all words that a fifth-grader can pronounce, understand, and recognize. In other words, 'butter' is easily said and understood, and someone can see that a stick of butter is butter. However, 'modified food starch,' though not too hard in the pronunciation department, doesn't actually mean anything to most people, and they certainly would not know if they saw a bag, stick, bucket (or whatever) of it.

Additives

Additives in general are bad news. You don't need to know much of anything about them individually if you don't want to; just stay away from them. An additive is something you put into a food not for 'food'-related reasons but for industrial reasons. Basically, if you don't recognize or know what a word is when you read it, you probably want to stay away from it.

Having said that, a lot of food products (especially rice, bread, and so on) are fortified with vitamins and minerals. These will show up in ingredient lists as strange-looking chemical names, but they're nothing to worry about. A list of common vitamins that get added to foods includes:

* **Thiamine**
* **Riboflavin**
* **Niacin**, Niacinamide
* **Biotin**
* **Folic Acid**
* **Ascorbic Acid**
* **Tocopherols**
* Pantothenic Acid
* Cyanocobalamin
* Pyridoxine
* Cholecalciferol
* Beta Carotene

This might seem like an intimidating list, but remember I'm not saying you need to memorize it, just be aware that there are some things that will show up in an ingredient list that aren't bad. You'll start to recognize them as you see them more and more, and I've bolded some of the more common ones.

Organic

Organic does not mean healthy. Organic just refers to the methods used to produce a food. It's a better option to buy the organic version of healthy food if the extra money makes no difference to you, but if money matters, it's much more important to buy healthy and natural food as opposed to processed food, even if you can't go for the organic version. There's organic soy oil, for example; it's still denatured and unhealthy. It's possible to eat an all-organic diet and still be very unhealthy, which cannot be said about a truly all-natural diet. Organic certainly isn't bad, but it's not enough on its own to make a food healthy.

It's important that you not see the cost of organic food as a barrier between you and a healthy diet, because you can be healthy without going organic.

P.S.

One thing worth noting here is that organic is a better option for fatty meats. Often, hormones and antibiotic residues get stored in fat, so fatty meats in particular are likely to have higher levels of these residues, which means if you're buying ribeye steaks or bacon, organic is a better choice than conventional.

Vitamins

Vitamins are extremely important, but you should get them from the source. It's not necessarily vital to know which vitamin is in which natural food AS LONG AS you eat an abundance of natural foods. Your body knows how to deal with vitamins in the context of the fruit or meat or other food they come in; it does not know what to do with vitamin pills (supplements). Eat natural foods in their natural state, and you will get plenty of vitamins!

Let me clarify here that I'm not going to tell anyone not to take a vitamin supplement, I simply want to emphasize that the best way to get vitamins is always when those vitamins occur naturally in the food you eat. If you do take a multivitamin supplement, think of it is a backup plan, not a primary strategy. Your primary concern with vitamins should always be to get an abundance of them, each day, from real foods.

Antioxidants

These are similar to vitamins and additives in that it is not important to know each one; an abundance of one specific antioxidant will not save you from yourself, no matter what any commercial for ketchup or some supplement tries to tell you. Natural, intact foods are full of viable antioxidants. Never believe anything that has 'added' antioxidants because in general antioxidants are far too fragile to isolate and then add to a food—remember that these antioxidants are ultimately added for marketing reasons, not for health reasons.

MSG

MSG (monosodium glutamate) is a notorious flavoring agent and probable neurotoxin responsible for a lot of upset stomachs, headaches, and other miscellaneous complaints. It is hidden under many names in many foods, particularly canned soups (so much so that I would avoid canned soups altogether). Many food items which boast about having no MSG contain other versions of it. Some other names include disodium inosinate, 'autolyzed' or 'hydrolyzed' anything, any kind of protein concentrate or protein isolate, any kind of modified starch, any kind of yeast extract or protein extract. Avoid these and the foods that contain them.

Fake Sugars

These include Splenda, Nutrasweet, aspartame, sucralose, acesulfame potassium, and so on. Don't ever eat them. What they do and where they go in your body is very poorly understood, and they completely disrupt your natural ability to crave healthy foods. Don't eat them. Healthy sweeteners include raw honey and raw agave nectar, should you need them. If you hate those and you absolutely have to use something, just add some normal sugar. As long as you don't go overboard, it's not the end of the world.

Never fall for 'natural' as a marketing tool. Develop an understanding for what this word actually means, and ignore it in any advertisement or on any packaging until you've checked it out for yourself.

Resources:

A Consumer's Dictionary of Food Additives, 7th Edition: Descriptions in Plain English of More Than 12,000 Ingredients Both Harmful and Desirable Found in Foods
By Ruth Winter

This is a great resource for anyone who is curious about those long words they always see in lists of ingredients and wonder just what they are and where they come from. Again, it's not necessary to know what every additive is and does, but it can be interesting to read up on some of them, and it's nice to have a comprehensive reference book like this at hand.

CRAVINGS

You've probably noticed by now that I'm a huge believer in the idea that your body is a way more sophisticated, impressive, effective machine than we give it credit for in the modern world—and that everything it does, it does for a reason—and that we'd all be better off if we'd just stop trying to fight it and learn to work with it. I don't believe this because I want to believe it, but because I've seen it in action and I know it to be true.

That should naturally give rise to more than a few questions, since this is a rather complicated situation. One of the big ones is probably "If my body is so smart and perfect, why do I crave food that is unhealthy for me? Why does my body seem to tell me to eat chocolate cake and drink orange soda? What gives?"

That's a perfectly valid question, and it's something we need to discuss. Understanding this is critical during the first two to four weeks after you eliminate unhealthy, unnatural foods from your diet, because at that point you will still be tempted back to your old lifestyle.

Consider animals in the wild. Does a lioness need to convince her cubs to eat meat the way a human mother convinces her children to eat broccoli? No. Every wild living thing on Earth eats exactly what it needs to survive. You don't find the odd rabbit who just has to eat meat, even though his body can't handle it, or the shark who only wants to eat seaweed and dies because of it. Wild animals eat what they love to eat, which is exactly what their bodies need—just watch them. They're not forcing it down.

When your body isn't full of the damaged nutrients that are standard in a modern diet, it will tell you what it needs and you will hear it, loud and clear. But when you're used to consuming preservatives, artificial sweeteners, food dyes, and other miscellaneous chemicals and synthetic 'foods,' your body becomes confused.

When you eat an apple, for example, your body has an innate ability to understand the value of the various components of that apple, and when you need them again, it will point you in that direction. However, when you eat packaged, processed apple sauce, something else happens. It's like eating an apple, but not really. Some things are damaged, some things are missing.

Your body doesn't get what it needs, and it tells you to keep looking—to keep eating. Since fruit (which is obviously very sweet) should be a major component of the human diet, and since few people eat anywhere near the amount of fresh fruit they should eat, many people are constantly craving sweets, and can't kill that craving no matter what, because they don't understand it.

When you mix in cheese crackers and chips and cake and soda and candy and diet foods and all the rest of it, so many foods with such artificially strong flavors and so little nutrient value, your natural inclination to crave what your body actually needs doesn't stand a chance. That's why many people just kind of want to eat everything, all the time, and no matter what they eat they still don't feel satisfied, because they never get the nutrients they're looking for.

I will say that I for one have very little self-control when it comes to food, but I don't need any. I eat as many grapes or as much watermelon or as much cheese or nuts or steak as I want. Because my cravings are in line with my body's needs, and because I don't confuse my body by giving it artificial flavorings and industrial additives and so on, that's exactly what I should be doing. You can get there too—anyone can—it just takes a level of understanding and self-control in the beginning.

If you don't believe me that your body will tell you to eat what it needs, look at pregnant women. Pregnant women, even those who don't steer clear of unnatural foods (which is most people in general), are in a heightened state of clarity as far as what their bodies need because they are in such an extreme biological situation. When their bodies are going through the process of actually creating another entire person, there are all kinds of nutrients they must use of types and in quantities that are very different from those normally required.

That's why they all get sudden, urgent cravings for all kinds of bizarre foods and food combinations—even though the women couldn't name the exact chemicals, proteins, vitamins, or whatever else they need, their bodies intuitively know where they are located and how to get them.

Most people only experience that kind of feeling when pregnant because the circumstances are extreme and the body is more or less able to cut through the fog created by all the chemicals and damaged elements of the modern diet. But the potential for that clarity is there for everyone, men and women, on a daily basis, if you just know how to access it.

This is where exercise comes in to the cravings equation (this will be discussed in more practical terms in the chapter that discusses the interaction between nutrition and exercise). After you exercise, your body must repair itself. It will crave certain things that it would not necessarily crave if you hadn't exercised. This situation is not nearly so pronounced as the one that occurs with a pregnant woman, but it does heighten your cravings to an extent.

For that reason, regular strenuous exercise is a great way to keep yourself 'on track' as far as understanding and responding correctly to your cravings, because it makes them stronger and easier to follow. Also, if you fall off the wagon and eat badly for a few days, you will feel worse while you exercise and you will take longer to recover afterward, which will train you on a conscious as well as subconscious level to avoid unnatural foods.

Basically, regular exercise will heighten the negative results of unhealthy eating, which will make unhealthy eating less and less pleasant and teach your body to crave only what will nourish it.

Although we think of cravings as something we should fight, in reality a craving tells you that your body needs something. Get used to satisfying cravings with natural foods—fresh ripe fruit, nuts, dairy, meat, etc.

I'm not saying that the next time you want candy you should just eat an apple and your desire for candy will completely disappear—most people have a lifetime of associating that sweet urge with candy/pastries/soda/whatever, and it doesn't go away instantly. However, I am saying that if you're strict with yourself for two weeks, add a lot of fresh fruit to your diet, and snack on fresh fruit instead of sweets when you're hungry, that urge for candy or cookies or chocolate or whatever else will be significantly reduced.

Learn to listen to your body. It's good at what it does.

CLEANSING

A lot of the difficulty people have with health comes from misinformation, and since there's a lot of talk lately about 'cleansing' and various cleansing products, I figured I'd talk about that a little bit.

First of all, the body has a tremendous ability to cleanse itself. There are a lot of processes that go on in your body in order for it to cleanse itself and it's not necessary to understand every single part of that, but basically cells clean themselves of toxins and when fresh blood comes through, the blood takes the toxins away to your kidneys, which clean out your blood.

So, your body does have an amazing capacity to clean itself, but it isn't really able to do this if it's hard at work digesting all the time. That's why it's a really bad idea to eat small meals all day long, because then you're digesting all day long and your body never gets the chance to clean itself (for our purposes, think of typical digestion and cleansing as two mutually exclusive things—not precisely true, but effectively true).

This is another reason why eating raw foods with useful enzymes and intact nutrients is so important. Eating fresh fruit isn't hard on your digestive system at all; in fact, it's very easy. So eating fruit doesn't get in the way of your body cleansing itself. But eating a lot of cooked and processed foods is really bad because not only are you putting damaged nutrients into your body that will need to be cleaned out, you're simultaneously making it more difficult for your body to do that cleaning by forcing it to undergo the difficult process of digesting that damaged food.

There are many types of 'cleansing' things you can do, and I can't possibly cover all of them (nor would that be useful). But here are a few pieces of advice.

1. You do not need any type of special product to cleanse yourself. Only trust a cleanse that uses real food (actual berries, not berry juice; actual fruit, not vitamin supplements, actual apple cider vinegar, not some prepackaged concoction containing it, etc.). Do not buy a special cleansing pill or potion with processed ingredients; you're wasting your time and your money.

2. Circulation is an incredible way to cleanse yourself. Blood cells are like little maintenance teams that go around your body cleaning up debris. The more rounds they make, the cleaner things are. So go on regular walks, breathe fresh air (and breathe deeply), and engage in regular exercise to increase circulation. This is a great way to keep your body clean all the time.

3. If your body is weary from digestion, it isn't cleansing. It's a good idea to have a breakfast that's just fruit, because it's very easy on your body and doesn't interrupt the cleaning your body has been going through since dinner last night. If you really want to cleanse yourself, consider spending an entire day, or a few days, eating nothing but as much fresh fruit, of any kind, as you want.

4. If you do some type of cleanse, especially if you haven't done it before, prepare to feel bad. During the cleanse, all of those toxins will get dumped into your blood stream, and until they get cleaned out you might feel pretty weak and nauseous. Plan accordingly.

5. Sweating is another great way to get toxins out of your blood stream. I had a professor who was a specialist in mushrooms and fungi, and he was called in when a patient at the local hospital who had overdosed on psychoactive mushrooms just wasn't getting better—months after his overdose, he was still weak, shaky, and sickly. Even though he had been on countless powerful drugs designed to clean out his system, he still had the toxins in his body. My professor took him off all medication, and told him to get a job in construction. Two weeks of hard, sweaty work later, he was almost back to normal. Simply sweating regularly can keep your body clean and efficient—and not ever sweating can mean a buildup of waste products and other toxins. Exercise regularly.

DIET AND EXERCISE

Understanding and appreciating this chapter could dramatically increase the results you get from this new way of understanding diet, exercise, and nutrition.

When people want to get healthier or change their lifestyles for the better, there are some who are more inclined to change their diets but not become more active, whereas others are more inclined to start exercising, but not do a whole lot from a nutritional standpoint.

Few people understand that once you get on the right track with the whole diet and exercise thing, employing these two things together can be the difference, in the long term, between failure and success.

Let's consider the person who exercises well but does not eat well. In this case, we will say that 'not eating well' generally means eating a lot of processed, damaged foods which are difficult for your body to digest and which introduce a lot of toxins that have to be cleaned from your bloodstream.

Well, if you exercise a lot, that means you will increase your circulation, which means that your blood will stop by your cells to pick up their waste. Since you don't eat too well, there will be a lot of waste products for them to pick up and then carry into your blood stream to be cleaned out.

This will make you feel like crap pretty much whenever you exercise, and obviously that's going to make it more difficult to do it regularly. Also, it will take you much longer to recover from exercise because your body won't have access to the best foods that you need to rebuild your body, and because it will be busy clearing out waste.

Let's look at the other side of the equation: what if you decide to eat well but not exercise? Well, eating the right foods and not putting toxins into your body is great, but the old, built-up toxins will take a while to get cleaned out because your circulation is never stimulated by exercise. Also, because you won't experience those heightened healthy cravings brought on by your body as it tries to recover from exercise, it will take more time for you to get into the routine of healthy eating, and it will be easier to fall out of it.

But let's look at what happens when you do both. Once you get into a routine of eating right (I mean really eating right, not what most people think is eating right) and exercising regularly, the two things really amplify each other. Because you eat well, you don't have to deal with a slew of toxins getting into your blood every time you exercise, which means you will work out more often and enjoy doing it. Also, your recovery time will be cut dramatically because your body will have access to all those important intact nutrients that most people never get.

Because you exercise, your circulating blood will regularly clean out your body and keep you free from toxins that cause nausea, fatigue, and other daily annoyances. Also, the recovery period after you exercise will help teach you instinctively to choose healthy, natural foods over the ones that are full of crap.

When you really understand what it means to eat well, and when you understand exactly how and why exercise is important, the two activities reinforce each other and deliver results significantly more impressive than either one alone. Further, either one alone is likely to be much more difficult to maintain because they are really two sides of the same issue. If you want the best results, you HAVE to incorporate both into your life. If you won't do that, there's not much I or anyone else can do for you.

Resources:

Natural Exercise: Basic Bodyweight Training and Calisthenics for Strength and Weight-Loss
By Patrick Barrett

Bodyweight exercises have been used by athletes and soldiers all over the world for many centuries. I wrote this book so that people would be able to learn everything they need to know about getting a full-body bodyweight workout, which includes information about breathing, joint development, rest and recovery, scheduling, and more, in addition to in-depth explanations and pictures of a highly effective core group of exercises.

BORN TO BE HEALTHY?

When a lot of mainstream nutrition and exercise 'experts' talk about how to be healthy, it almost sounds like you and your body are on opposing teams—your body wants to be fat and sedentary, and you have to find ways to trick it to be healthy.

It seems to me, though, that there is every indication that your body wants to be healthy, and the poor health that we see so frequently really comes from people not understanding what their bodies want and need, and not knowing how to give it to them.

Let's think about this for a moment, and let's assume, if only for the sake of argument, that your body is perfectly designed to be healthy. What does that mean?

Well, you have color vision so that you can recognize and evaluate brightly-colored fruits, as well as vegetables. Conversely, as fruits and vegetables ripen and reach the peak of flavor, the color becomes deeper, bolder, and more attractive to your eyes. You also have opposable thumbs for grasping and peeling fruit. Have you ever noticed how a lot of the healthiest foods—pomegranates, berries, and many other fruits and vegetables—are brightly colored? Just as bees can see wavelengths of light that we can't which help them to find the right flowers, we can see which parts of plants contain useful nutrients, especially when they are at their peak in flavor and nutrition.

And what about your nose and tongue? Think about it— what is the point, from a biological standpoint, of things tasting or smelling bad or good to us? It's so that you can find healthy food. Rocks don't taste good, so we don't eat them. Fruit does, so we do. I know there are unhealthy things that taste good too, but you need to remember that your body is something ancient living in a modern world —your nose and mouth are made to appreciate 'ancient' foods—foods that would have existed centuries or millenia ago—and if you stick to the ancient foods that taste and smell delicious, you won't go wrong. Fruit, vegetables, meat, nuts, dairy—these are all ancient foods. Soy bars, candy, pills and powders—these are distinctly not ancient.

You have a combination of flat teeth for processing vegetation, and sharp canine teeth for processing meat. You don't have a digestive tract that can effectively process raw grains. This is because both meat and vegetation are part of your body's ideal diet, and grains aren't. Your body is the way it is for a reason. I could write a lot more about this but I just want to get you away from the idea that your body is stupidly designed and built to break. It is not. If you can learn to appreciate how well-designed your body is, and how what's healthy for you actually makes sense, your whole perspective on maintaining and optimizing your health will change.

Realize that your body is good at what it does, and learn to listen to it in the right way.

ALKALINITY

A good way to understand the foods you consume is in terms of alkalinity and acidity. Body pH is extremely important. You could write a whole book on this subject, but suffice it to say that the types of foods you eat impact the pH of your intracellular fluids and other body fluids (not so much your blood, which must maintain a pretty narrow pH, or you die). Cooked and processed foods are pretty much universally acidifying—which is bad for your body, makes it difficult to clean out waste products, and sets the stage for chronic diseases like cancer (cancer requires an acidic environment to survive).

Raw fruit is alkalizing, which is extremely important, and another reason to consume a lot of fruit.

Determining whether a food makes your fluids more acidic or alkaline is not a simple matter of finding out the pH of the food itself, but a matter of understanding how the food is digested and metabolized. For example, orange juice itself is acidic, but fresh-squeezed orange juice is alkalizing, whereas pasteurized store-bought orange juice is acidifying.

To my knowledge, no one has tested to see if raw meat and raw dairy is acidifying or alkalizing, but cooked meat and dairy are acidifying. Generally speaking, protein sources are acidifying, which is okay as long as they're balanced by the alkalizing effects of a lot of raw, fresh fruit. If they aren't—and they aren't for most people—then nearly everything you eat is acidifying, which is very hard on your body when it comes to digestion, exercise, cleansing, and general well-being.

Coffee is not good for you. The high dose of caffeine is bad for you, and the coffee is highly acidifying. If you depend on it, wean yourself off. Green tea is better and will give you a reduced caffeine kick if you need it—but 'needing' caffeine is not a good strategy in general.

Use sea salt. It contains a much healthier balance of minerals, and in my opinion it tastes much better. When I first switched to sea salt I didn't really notice a difference, but now when I taste regular salt it tastes like chemicals to me, and I don't ever use it. Also, because of the additional minerals it contains, sea salt is alkalizing, whereas table salt is acidifying.

You don't have to find out the pH effect of everything you eat, but this is yet another interesting predictor of health which points to the 'natural' diet as an ideal solution.

Resources:

The Acid-Alkaline Food Guide: A Quick Reference to Foods & Their Effect on pH Levels
By Susan E. Brown and Larry Trivieri Jr.

This book gives a very concise and interesting presentation of the body pH argument, as well as a reference guide for the relative alkalinity of most common foods.

BREAKING YOUR PROCESSED CARBOHYDRATE ADDICTION

Processed carbohydrates are nothing short of an addiction. You must free yourself from this. Most people think of chips or pretzels or crackers or similar snack foods as an acceptable part of your diet. They really are not. It doesn't matter how many calories they contain or whether they're 'light' or 'diet' or whatever. You should start to think of all cookies, crackers, chips, pretzels, brownies, cake, and yes, even bread and pasta as part of the "processed carbohydrate" group, which is something you don't want to be a part of your regular diet.

This is not easy. I remember when I started to eat this way, the idea of not eating bread and pasta was very difficult. I was legitimately sad about it, like I was saying goodbye to an old friend. It was much harder, psychologically, than I thought it would be.

But it goes a lot easier than you think if you just commit to it in the beginning. First start by eliminating all those 'snack foods.' They're terrible for you, empty of all nutrition, and only make it more difficult for your body to do what it needs to do.

Then, begin to eat bread and pasta less and less frequently. Before long you'll notice how heavy and tired you feel after eating these foods, and you just won't feel like having them anymore—when you're used to the easier digestion of meals without a lot of processed grains, just the idea of eating a big bowl of pasta will put you right to sleep.

But take cutting out snack foods seriously. It's a huge deal.

NUTRITION IN THE MEDIA

One of the biggest obstacles standing between most people and ideal health is misinformation, and pretty much all of that misinformation comes to us through the media—that includes magazines, newspapers, commercials, the news, and so on. If you want to become, and stay, a healthy person, you need to learn how to deal with this.

In the modern world, a lot of people care about nutrition—they want to lose weight, be healthier, and live longer. Even unhealthy people who take no steps to become healthy still take note of nutrition news, which is why all these media outlets love to seize on any new story about some study or some theory about how people can lose weight and live longer—just like every new company with some pill or powder that's going to undo an unhealthy lifestyle is dying to get their 'news' out in front of the public.

Think about where your food information comes from. Don't believe commercials. More often than not if you get information about nutrition from the television or a magazine, whether it's an ad, a show, or an article, (even the news), somebody paid for it to be there and somebody is making money off of it. Most people don't think about it, but the majority of the ideas we have about health and nutrition come from commercials, and things printed on the label of the food itself. These people are not out to make you healthy or be your friend, they're out to make money.

That doesn't mean that everything you hear is a lie, but it does mean you should be skeptical of everything you hear. Don't believe claims until you've seen them in action and you know they're accurate. Eating healthy should make you feel good, and it doesn't require any unnatural food products. I would be very suspicious of anyone who tells you you need some kind of pill, powder, bar, or potion to stay healthy.

CONCLUSION

Whew! That's a lot of information. I know for a lot of you some of this comes as a surprise, and you may not be sure where to go from here. In this chapter I'd like to review, briefly, the information from the other chapters, and give you some more specific directions on your eating habits.

Most 'diets' will give you some level of pretty specific instructions. Either they will lay out exactly what meals you should eat and at what time, or they will single out some particular elements and tell you to eat at least, or no more than, a certain amount every day.

This is not a 'diet' in that sense. Those kinds of diets are stupid. This is intended to be a way to help you understand what your body needs to be healthy, all the time. I'm not going to tell you exactly what to eat, nor should anyone else who has never met you, because I don't know anything about you. My goal is to help you understand better how your body actually works, and which foods help it and which foods harm it. Once you know that, you need to make some of your own decisions and start paying attention to the impact they have on your day-to-day health and well-being.

Am I going to tell you not to eat in restaurants any more? No. Would that make you healthier? Probably. But going out with your friends and not being a pain in the ass about what you order isn't going to make or break you from a health standpoint. I eat out with friends, I even have fast food once in a while if I'm on the road or the people I'm with want to. So, you feel like crap and you don't do it again for a while—it's fine.

If you personally know that you should stay away from some things because you can't control yourself around them, then you need to be aware of them and act accordingly, but I won't pretend that that's a rule that applies to everybody. If you're not willing and able to 'know yourself' and take responsibility for the decisions you make, then I can't help you and neither can anybody else.

The biggest problem that people face when trying to lose weight, get in shape, and generally get healthy is that they don't actually know what's healthy, what's unhealthy, and why. Now you have a pretty good idea about all of those things. So what do you do?

The overwhelming piece of advice that you MUST follow is to eat natural foods. You probably 'knew' that before, but you didn't really understand what it actually meant, or why it was so important. You need to get into the habit of looking at the ingredient list on whatever you're thinking about buying. The best way to handle this is to get food from the butcher or the produce section, which has no ingredient list (because it's only one thing). That way, you can prepare it yourself and know exactly what you're eating. Otherwise, check to make sure that the food is free from unnatural fats, preservatives, additives, and chemicals.

In general, I like to eat fruit and dairy during the day and meat/fish and vegetables at night. You don't have to follow that schedule, you can figure out any one you like, but that works for me. I recommend one to three meals over the course of the day and as much fresh fruit at any time of the day or night as you feel like having.

As I said, this is my personal preference and you don't need to follow it exactly. If you're serious about improving your eating habits, getting in shape, and staying healthy for the rest of your life, I would say you need to follow these basic rules:

   1. Significantly reduce or eliminate regular consumption of cooked, processed carbohydrates.
   2. Stop eating unnatural fats.
   3. Eliminate unnatural additives and preservatives.
   4. Eat a lot of fruit.
   5. Eat protein.
   6. Drink water.

Those are the most important things. As far as sources of protein goes, go with whatever combination of meat, fish, eggs, nuts, beans, and dairy you like, as long as they fit the above criteria. Ideally, animal proteins would be as lightly cooked as possible, but if that freaks you out, it's not the end of the world.

In my experience, what's good for your body is simple and logical. Your body handles meat and animal fat and fruit really well because these are the things that we and our ancestors have been eating for millenia. Your body does not handle soy milk and vegetable seed oils and protein bars and cheese crackers and processed, pasteurized fruit products because these are all inventions of the past few decades that are totally foreign to it.

When you eat healthy, you should feel healthy and energized and light on your feet and just good. If you have heartburn or indigestion or fatigue or dry mouth or trouble sleeping or trouble concentrating or trouble recovering from exercise, your diet is wrong. That's all there is to it.

You now have a good handle on what it means to provide your body with the nutrients it needs, and to avoid damaged and toxic foods and food products. As you apply this knowledge to your daily life, remember to take notice of the various changes in your body—noticing improvements is what will keep you motivated to stay healthy.

RESOURCES

This is a master list of the resources mentioned at the end of the other chapters:

Natural Exercise: Basic Bodyweight Training and Calisthenics for Strength and Weight-Loss
By Patrick Barrett

The Whole Soy Story: The Dark Side of America's Favorite Health Food
By Kaayla T. Daniel

Ignore the Awkward: How the Cholesterol Myths Are Kept Alive
By Dr. Uffe Ravnskov

The Coconut Oil Miracle
By Bruce Fife and Jon J. Kabara

The Acid-Alkaline Food Guide: A Quick Reference to Foods & Their Effect on pH Levels

By Susan E. Brown and Larry Trivieri Jr.

A Consumer's Dictionary of Food Additives, 7th Edition: Descriptions in Plain English of More Than 12,000 Ingredients Both Harmful and Desirable Found in Foods
By Ruth Winter

The Untold Story of Milk: The History, Politics and Science of Nature's Perfect Food
By Ron Schmid

ABOUT THE AUTHOR

Patrick Barrett has been interested in exercise ever since he started to lift weights with his dad and older brothers as a kid. He participated in a half-dozen organized sports (most notably inline hockey and high school wrestling) until a neck injury during a wrestling match in his junior year prevented him from playing further in any contact sports.

After the injury, he developed an interest in pursuing strength and balance, particularly through bodyweight and self-taught gymnastic-type exercises.

Patrick has always loved both cooking and eating food. Unsatisfied with the confusing and often contradictory nutritional advice offered by mainstream sources, Patrick searched for another way to understand human nutrition that was logical, consistent, and effective. His books on food and nutrition reflect this 'cleaner,' more intuitive and useful understanding of food and how it impacts our health.

Patrick hopes that his books will save his audience time and aggravation by finally offering practical ways to achieve their nutrition and fitness goals.

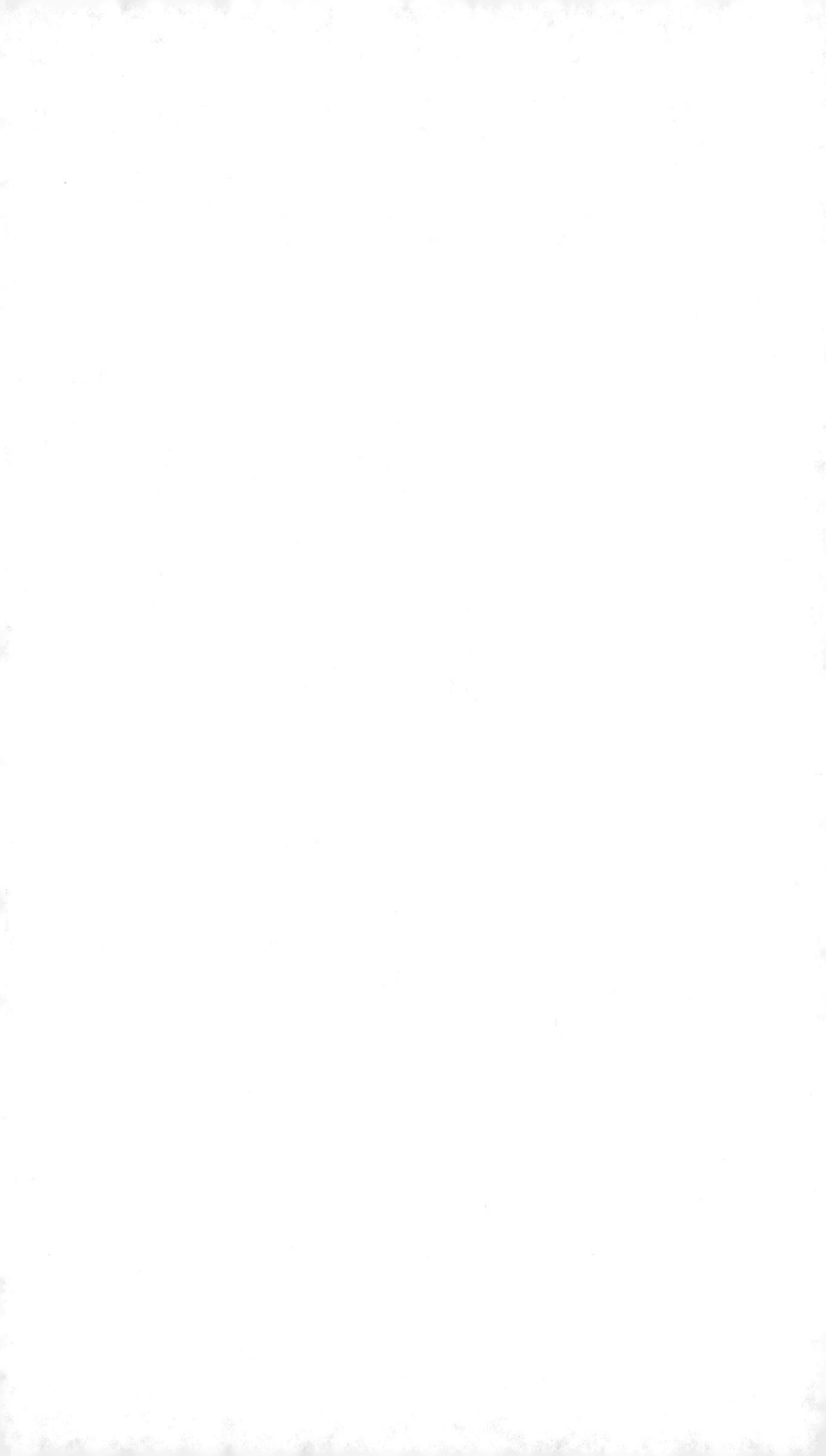